THE HEART OF THE KEY TO CANCER

THE HEART OF
THE KEY TO CANCER

What we understand, we can deal with

[handwritten inscription and signature]

Richard S. Weeder, M.D. FACS,
President, Richard Weeder Cancer
Education Foundation

Ian Okazaki, M.D.
Hawai'i Pacific Health
Straub Medical Center
Division of Hematology/Oncology
Honolulu, Hawaii

*The spiritual power of Eastern practices
linked to the scientific rigor of Western
medical research is potent therapy.*

RWCancer.org

Contents

Dedication

To the loving memory of Harry Croft Bickel and Zachary Arnold Simpson, M.D., FACS. Both men of character whose lives illuminated those around them.

Acknowledgments

First and foremost, to Dr. Dean Ornish, who has done for heart disease what we are attempting with cancer. His program and ideas have been an inspiration and an influence on our own.

To Paracelsus and Sir William Osler who, in their times, changed the course of medicine.

To the late Prof. Malcolm Diamond, mentor and friend at Princeton, whose influence is found in chapter two. And to my premedical advisor at Princeton, Dr. Allen O. Whipple.

To my mentors in surgery: my father, S. Dana Weeder M.D., and those at Penn—Drs. I. S. Ravdin, Jonathan E. Rhoads, and C. Everett Koop. At Geisinger Medical Center, I owe a debt to Drs. Harold Foss, Harry Klinger, and Frank Gerow.

To my brother and brother-in-law, Dana N. Weeder M.D. and Zachary A. Simpson M.D., who cleared a path for me to follow in the profession.

To my friends and colleagues on The Islands. To Drs. Frank Tabrah, Fedor Lurie, James McKoy, Laeton Pang and Charles Miller. To Ira Zunin M.D., President, the Hawaii State Consortium for Integrative Healthcare. To Corinne and Nathan Shulman, for steady encouragement and good advice. To our webmaster, Norman Miller, for sharing the intricacies of computers and making it seem easy. To all of you, mahalo, and keep up the good work.

To my wife and best editor, Areta Oebel Parlé, for good counsel and support without limits.

R. S. Weeder

DISCLAIMER

Mark Twain advised, "Beware of reading medical books; you may die of a misprint." Such is not likely with this book as it is meant to be educational rather than a source of medical advice. Medical advice should always come from your physician, and any ideas you may pick up from us should be cleared with your physician.

Introduction

"Dick Weeder has been an innovative thinker and leader
in recognizing the role of immunity in health. He is
passionately dedicated to teach cancer patients to increase
their innate immunity through non-traditional pathways
as a complement traditional care. The most recent edition
of *Key to Cancer* is a guide for patient empowerment and
is more pertinent today than originally conceived."
Joseph Carver, M.D. University of Pennsylvania.

This book is written for the cancer patient. It is particularly written
for the patient whose cancer is out of control.

Now we have all heard stories about cancer patients who
far outlived a dire prognosis: their cases are variously labeled
"spontaneous remissions," "remarkable recoveries," and "miracle
cures." This book describes how these "miracles" are possible for you,
but from a scientific point of view and without divine intervention.

The crux of the matter is that cancer is not the cause of the
disease, but a symptom of an underlying problem. And, like treating
a fever instead of the infection causing it, most of us have been
treating only the effect (tumor), unaware that a cause lies behind it.
Doctors dislike complex treatments; simplicity is an ideal. But it is

1

increasingly apparent that cancer is highly complex, and the sooner we accept this reality, the sooner we will treat cancer adequately. This book will suggest that those who have remarkably recovered have discovered for themselves the need to treat the disease in all its complexity.

Parenthetically, in the last thirty years, there have been two major advances in medicine, both involving a shift in treatment from the effect of a disease to its cause. In heart disease, we started unblocking the arteries that had injured the muscle. In peptic ulcer disease, one doctor, Barry Marshall, recognized that an ulcer is caused by a bacterium in the tissues beneath it and simply treated the ulcer with an antibiotic. In both instances, a conceptual shift from effect to cause led to dramatic improvements in results. We believe that this shift in focus will provide the same improved results with cancer. Early experience has begun to bear this out.

It seems that, from birth, we are protected from cancer (and a lot of other conditions) by a "protective complex" of immunity, energy-related resources, and many factors that may be included in the category "spirit" or will. These latter include optimism, faith, curiosity, joy, laughter, relationships and many other unmeasurable gifts.

The chapters which follow will go more deeply into our thesis and will then provide effective tools for you to strengthen your protective complex. Thus educated, you will know how to treat your cancer, both cause and effect. What one truly understands, one can deal with.

1

A Second Look at Cancer

Thesis: We believe that cancer is not the cause of illness but rather a lapse in the complex mechanisms of immunity, energy, and spirit that ordinarily protect us.

This idea explains many of the mysteries of advanced cancer. And a shift in thinking may suggest important aspects of both treatment and prevention. We are speaking primarily of advanced cancer that has not been fully destroyed by surgery, chemotherapy, and/or radiotherapy. We have all witnessed many or all of these mysteries:

1. Uneven response to therapy among those with similar tumors and stages
2. Long term remissions with unexplained relapses.
3. The increased rate of malignancy in immune-deficiency disease (AIDS).
4. Inaccuracy in predictions of life expectancy for those with advanced disease.
5. The appearance, or reappearance, of cancer following a stressful life experience.
6. The unexplained "spontaneous remission," "remarkable recovery," or "miracle cure," whatever you wish to name it.

7. The idea that the average seventy-year old has had a few cancers during that life span, most or all of which never became clinically apparent. Cancer seems a constant, dormant threat, like the flu and the common cold.

8. Treatment and outcome frequently seem unconnected, as if there is an unexplained intervening factor.

9. Most cancer patients who are not cured leave us by a common pathway of loss of weight, loss of energy, and loss of spirit or hope.

10. The case of the light smoker who gets lung cancer and the heavy smoker who does not.

Cancer can be visualized as if on one side of a scale, with the Protective Complex on the other side (See Figure 1). Which way the scale swings determines the outcome.

Figure 1

TUMOR	vs.	ENERGY
		IMMUNITY
		WILL

Figure 2
Protective Complex

Immunity	Energy (Chi)	Spirit (will to live)
The Immune System	Exercise	Meditation
Massage	Nutrition	Relationships
Acupuncture	Yoga/Tai Chi	Attitude/Optimism
Exercise	Oxygen	Philosophy/faith
Pos. Attitude (Psycho-neuroimmunology)	Rest	Laughter, Usefulness, Music, Arts, Hobbies

For the purposes of simplifying discussion, and throughout the book, I am going to refer to the medical therapy provided by M.D.s and D.O.s, and usually rendered in hospitals, as "Western Medicine." This is also labeled "Conventional Medicine." For the modalities and techniques commonly called "Complementary," "Integrative," "Alternative," or "Eastern" (Chinese), I have used the term "CAM" (complementary-alternative medicine) therapy. Neither of these labels is perfect, but I believe most readers will be familiar with their use.

Figure 2 describes the factors which make up the Protective Complex. There may be other factors not listed. And while many of these modalities influence immunity, we should still consider them therapeutically one by one. They are listed in no particular order of importance.

Figure 3 lists various therapeutic modalities, points out where they usually operate, and shows if their influence is positive, negative, or neutral (**O**) with regard to the protective complex. The list is by no means complete.

Figure 3

	Less Tumor Burden	Immunity	Energy	Hope	Less Pain
EXERCISE	O	+	+	+	O
MASSAGE	O	+	+	+	O
ACUPUNCTURE	O	+	+	+	+
MEDITATION	O	+	+	+	+
CHEMOTHERAPY, RADIOTHERAPY, SURGERY	+	neg.	neg.	+	+
NUTRITION, ANTIOXIDANTS	+	+	+	+	O
ATTITUDINAL HEALING	O	+	+	+	O
YOGA	O	+	+	+	+

A parallel with the treatment of heart disease is clear. For the first three quarters of the last century, we treated heart attacks by focusing on the injured muscle, using mostly medications and virtually ignoring the primary defect in the coronary arteries. A little like tuning up a car engine while its fuel line is partly blocked! Then a surgical resident in Cleveland (Rene Favoloro) began repairing the vessels and the paradigm for treating heart disease shifted from effect to cause and surgeons became close colleagues with cardiologists in the care of heart disease. This was followed by Dean Ornish's careful work on reopening partly blocked vessels with diet, exercise, stress management and support group reinforcement—a further, broad based attack on the cause rather than the effect.

A similar phenomenon occurred in the treatment of peptic ulcers. Dr. Barry Marshall suggested that ulcers were usually caused by an infection in the tissues beneath the ulcer. Again, therapeutic attention was refocused from effect to cause, antibiotics were prescribed, and the ulcers healed.

Our approach to cancer up to now has primarily utilized Western Medicine, virtually ignoring the long medical traditions of China and the East. Yet these practitioners have developed a system of care that uses effective botanicals, acupuncture, and an understanding of energy, or Chi. They have much to offer us, and cancer is big enough and complex enough that we need all the help we can get. It is far more complex than heart disease or ulcer, whose origins are much more straightforward.

I have enormous respect for my oncologist colleagues, struggling to keep abreast of exploding knowledge in both chemotherapy and radiation therapy, meanwhile treating patients with great care and compassion. But they cannot and should not be asked to become expert in the foreign terrain of CAM (complementary alternative medicine) therapy.

Figure 4 is perhaps the most interesting of all. This curve is familiar to every oncologist, and it applies to every type of cancer known. It reveals how there are a few patients who "beat the odds" and become "spontaneous remissions," "miracle cures," and long-term survivors. We believe these few have discovered how to repair their "Protective Complexes," either knowingly or instinctively. No oncologist, I believe, would maintain that his or her modality can destroy every last nest of tumor cells in a patient with metastatic disease. In our view, the P. C., if healthy, acts as the "mop-up crew," to finish the job started by surgery, chemotherapy and radiotherapy. This leaves the patient to survive, effectively tumor-free.

Figure 4

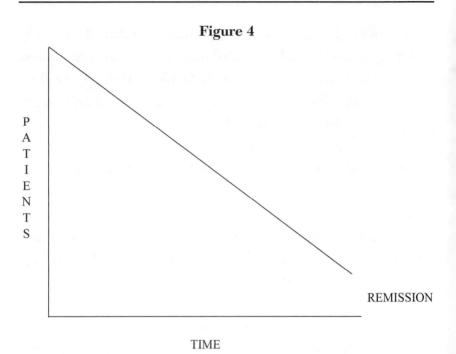

The area of "spirit" or will to live has often been derided by our more scientific-minded colleagues, who are unmoved by anything "unprovable." Paracelsus, five hundred years ago, stated, "Diseases come from the realm of Nature; healing comes from the realm of Spirit." No seasoned oncologist would deny the importance of will to live in a cancer patient, and the discipline known as psychoneuroimmunology (connecting thought, endocrine secretion and the immune system) has established its scientific validity.

WHY DID I GET CANCER?

This may be the most frequent question patients ask their doctors. For the long-term smoker, the light-skinned sun worshipper, the person with a genetic predisposition, the answer may be obvious. But for the majority, the answer is complex. As we have suggested, it is a defect in the Protective Complex. Maybe you can answer your own question by reviewing the number of factors in your life that may have injured either immunity, energy resources, your spirit, or a combination of all three. Ours is a complex answer to a simple question, but one that you can do something about.

With our thesis, we have adhered to a primary principle in medicine—to treat the cause before the effect, the infection before the fever. Whenever doctors have done otherwise, treatment has fallen short. Our answer implies educational and therapeutic collaborations such as we have never before tried. But it will surely lead to improved survival as well as better quality of life for the patient. Hopefully, it will also lead to more personal, more "tailor made" care. But how this new paradigm will work out between healers of many modalities is the subject of the rest of the book.

2

A Short Course on Cancer

HOW DOES CANCER WORK?

The development of clinically important cancer, cancer serious enough to make us sick, occurs because of a multitude of factors, a complex causality. It has been shown that we are all fighting off cancer throughout our lifetimes. If one draws blood from a "healthy" person, one often finds malignant cells present in the specimen. And the estimate has been made that every individual who lives out a normal life span has had an average of six cancers during that time, most of them, of course, not evident to the individual. So if we are frequently fighting off cancers, why do some become apparent and threaten our lives?

Some of the factors that operate in the development of malignancies include chronic irritants, decreased immunity, genetic predisposition, and fatigue, or loss of energy. Chronic irritants include such factors as inhaled particles (e.g. cigarette smoke) in the lungs, excessive sunlight to the skin, and fluctuating hormones (breast, prostate, uterine and ovarian cancer). Various ingested chemicals can affect the urinary bladder, and fatty acids from meat breakdown can stimulate cancer in the large intestine. What apparently happens is that, as the tissues attempt to heal themselves from this chronic damage, rapidly growing cells "de-differentiate" into out-of-control malignant cells.

Our exposure to chronic irritants is something we can usually control. One can avoid cigarette smoke, excessive sunlight, and unhealthy diets. Enough said. Genetics, as of this writing, may be harder to deal with, although there is promising research into this factor. What this little book will deal with, in some detail, are four factors: tumor destruction, immunity enhancement, energy stores and spiritual resilience. But first we will deal with how best to approach the threat of a malignancy.

CANCER AND ATTITUDE

I was lucky to have as friend and mentor Professor Malcolm Diamond of the Religion Department of Princeton University. He was one of my favorite teachers; in later years he became a close friend and valued mentor. One day at lunch I asked him, in all his experience with the world's great scriptures, what passage had the most meaning for him personally. He answered not from the Bible, the Torah, or the Tao Te Ching, but from *Lord Jim*, by Joseph Conrad. The passage is as follows. Stein and Marlow are having a philosophical talk about life, and Stein remarks:

> *"A man that is born falls into a dream like a man who falls into the sea. If he tries to climb out, as inexperienced people endeavor to do, he drowns—nicht wahr... No! I tell you! The way is to the destructive element submit yourself; and with the exertions of your hands and feet in the water make the deep, deep sea keep you up.*

Ever since Mal shared this passage with me, I have felt it to be the perfect metaphor for how to deal with cancer. Particularly for a swimmer somewhat afraid of the water, I appreciate the idea that one does not flail about but rather immerses oneself, gently but firmly stroking, and thus survives. So, my advice is to find out as much as you can about cancer and its cures, immerse yourself in the destructive element, as it were. Neither give up on the one extreme, nor panic on the other. Keep your "cool," your equanimity. Like a confrontation that you have dreaded, screw up your courage and enter it, fully prepared, head up. You may or may not be "cured." As another friend of mine says, "We none of us get out of here alive." But you have increased your chances of cure, and prolonged your useful life in the meantime. Become a "swimmer of the deep", and you will do well.

A PANORAMIC VIEW OF CURE

Now how does one get rid of cancer? First and foremost is the removal of the tumor mass by means of surgery, chemotherapy, and/or radiotherapy. These techniques lower the "tumor burden" by decreasing the number of malignant cells. And, though certainly the first and perhaps the most important measures in treating cancer, they are far from being the only things we can do.

During my medical school years I worked with Dr. C. Everett Koop, later to become famous as Surgeon General under President Reagan. Dr. Koop and I studied the neuroblastoma, a malignant tumor in children which has the unusual propensity to routinely disappear after it has been only partially removed. This "spontaneous remission" is a phenomenon that has been witnessed in every cancer known to medical science, although with far less regularity than is the case with neuroblastoma. This is the reason for so-called "Miracle cures," where a malignant tumor is cured without treatment. But in the case of neuroblastoma, what apparently happens is that, with the removal of part of the tumor, the tumor burden is lowered enough so that the child's natural defenses are able to eradicate the remainder. In the case of spontaneous remission without surgery or other treatment, presumably something has happened to strengthen the patient's defenses to the point of attacking and destroying the tumor. It does, indeed, seem miraculous. And yet, in truth, I believe such extraordinary cures are accessible to many of us if we broaden our present way of dealing with cancer.

The immune system is one of three other major factors which control cancers. Parenthetically, AIDS is such a devastating condition because it cripples the immune system, resulting in lowered resistance to both infections and malignancies. It should be noted that not all tumors are "malignant;" a malignant tumor being characterized not only by overgrowth of cells but by continued local or distant growth to the point where the tumor becomes metabolically draining and energy-depleting (which may be different aspects of the same thing.) Not so a benign tumor, which, although it may grow slowly to a very large size, remains localized. And it is through this distant growth or unrestrained growth at the original site that a malignant tumor makes such a drain on the patient's reserves.

The next important aspect of malignancy is the energy loss which it represents. Although hard to measure, our energy reserves are what make all activities possible. In the face of great energy loss, or fatigue, the resistance to a malignant tumor becomes nearly impossible.

Lastly, we recognize the emotional or spiritual aspect of cancer. This may be described as will-to-live, optimism, attitude, motivation, faith, call it what you will. But without it, all therapy is doomed. As Sören Kierkegaard said, "despair is the sickness unto death."

THE ADVANCES OF CONVENTIONAL MEDICAL THERAPY

The conventional treatment of cancer has been one of the great success stories of modern medicine. Although far from eradicated, cancer is certainly more effectively treated than it used to be. Surgery, the earliest form of treatment, remains most effective for many types of tumor: breast, lung, colon, skin, and brain, to name a few. For early, localized, cases, it is often enough to simply remove sufficient tumor so that few if any tumor cells remain, leaving any residual for the immune system to deal with.

Chemotherapy has become increasingly effective in the treatment of malignancies. Its value varies with the type of tumor treated; some malignancies are eradicated with up to 100% success, others less effectively. But with every passing year, more types of malignancy are coming under the control of an increasing array of chemical agents. And along with this increasing potency has come greater sophistication in avoiding the complications of chemotherapy.

Radiotherapy has also made great strides in cancer therapy, offering a variety of modalities either alone or in combination with chemotherapy and surgery. It goes without saying that modern cancer care involves a decision to use some or all of the above, as indicated by the tumor in question. All may be seen, in their effects, as decreasing the "tumor burden," the drain of energy which, left unchecked, may result in death.

Now one may ask how these therapies will preserve energy and life when they are all, to one extent or another, energy drains themselves. The answer lies in the fact that all are more damaging to tumor cells than they are to normal cells. Certainly, surgical operations take a toll in strength and nutrition. But physically removing the tumor does more good than harm. And, by the same token, chemotherapy and radiotherapy destroy more cancer cells than they do normal ones. Contrary to popular belief, cancer cells are weak and disorganized; they do their damage by their enormous drain of reserves through unrestrained proliferation. Chemotherapy and radiation attack rapidly growing cells, of which cancer cells are the most rapidly growing. Other rapidly growing cells are in the blood-forming areas (bone marrow), gut lining (mouth to anus), and hair follicles—thus the well-known chemotherapy side effects of hair loss, sore mouth, nausea, diarrhea, and anemia. But, again, the patient may take comfort in the fact that the tumor is being damaged more than his or her mucous membranes, bone marrow, and hair follicles. I tell my patients to look at each lost hair as a gravestone for five dead cancer cells. They feel much better about it.

So this battle with cancer can be considered like a contest on a see-saw or a balance scale, with the tumor on one side and the person's defenses on the other (see chapter 1). Surgery, radiotherapy, and chemotherapy are removing tumor burden, favorably altering the balance. But, on the other hand, there are things one can do to improve the other three factors: immunity, energy resources and will to live. They add weight and swing the balance in the direction of health. So let's discuss these other measures which are particularly useful for those patients whose tumors are advanced.

The immune system, very briefly, functions as follows. There are groups of white blood cells, specifically "T" cells and "NK" (natural killer) cells, which destroy foreign cells and material, removing them from the body. Now cancer cells may be recognized as foreign, so they are attacked and destroyed. The number of this army of T and NK cells is affected by a whole array of factors, so these factors become important in cancer resistance. Such factors include rest, nutrition, stress, grief, excess sugar, exercise, and massage. (For a detailed discussion of Immunity, see *The Road to Immunity*, by Kenneth Bock, M.D. and Nellie Sabin.) Use of antioxidants may encourage cellular immunity, but should be used with caution if you are undergoing chemotherapy. (The antioxidants may protect the cancer cells as well as the good ones.) Likewise, use massage with care, particularly in the area around a malignancy or if you have a weakened bone. Aromatherapy may be useful, particularly in conjunction with hot baths and before trying to sleep.

Bock describes in detail supplements which boost the immune system. These include vitamins C, B complex, A, E, Beta Carotene and the carotenoids. I refer you to his book mentioned above for a complete listing of these substances.

I particularly like to think of cancer in terms of energy stores. To imagine it visually, consider that we have a bucket of available energy. Cancer is a large hole in the bottom of the bucket. Surgery, radiotherapy and chemotherapy slow the drainage but are themselves energy drains. There are other, completely positive, ways to add energy to our bucket, such as getting rid of a chronic worry. This will have a direct inhibiting effect on the cancer.

Nicholas Gonzales, M.D. from New York advocates a complex nutritional and metabolic approach to pancreatic cancer and claims good results. I believe that nutrition and energy are two sides of the same coin, two ways of looking at the same thing. And the immune system is dependent on both. Certainly, the last word is yet to be written on the treatment of cancer. But, as the disease has many causal aspects, affects many organs, it seems likely that more cures will result when many modalities are used. Cancer is, unquestionably, a physical disease, with physical and environmental causes. It is a disease of the individual organ, but also a failure of the immune system. It is an energy "wasting" disease, like a major burn. And it is a disease having both roots and effects in the patient's spirit. I think it is only by addressing all these aspects that we will have great success in its treatment.

SPIRIT AND CANCER

Let us look more deeply into the spiritual or attitudinal aspect. When we are first told, "you have cancer," our perception is that we have been attacked from inside. It is not an outside blow, with a broken arm the result. Nor is it an invading bacteria. No, this is our own body threatening us, becoming our enemy. Imagine the sense of betrayal felt by a woman with breast cancer. What was previously a source of pride, of sexual attractiveness and prowess, an object of intimacy with lover and child, a source of nourishment for baby, has now become the agent of disease and possible death. What anguish and despair must arise from such an awful transformation.

Note the interrelationship with energy. If one is depressed, threatened, or anxious, energy leaks out of us from every pore. And cancer is certainly a great enough threat to cause depression and anxiety. Psychoneuroimmunology has demonstrated the indirect but undeniable link between what we think, the endocrine system and the immune system.

There are several things I use to raise my spirits. Creating something new always helps, whether the creation is intellectual or artistic. Likewise, exercise usually helps—the body seems to invigorate the spirit as it does the muscles—perhaps through endorphins. "Learned optimism," as advocated by Martin Seligman, is certainly a useful concept. As I've grown older, I've come to rely on meditation and Yoga—my day doesn't start without them. The word "Yoga" means yoke, and I like to think I'm yoking my mind, body and spirit together while I'm going through the postures. It's a little like making the connections between ignition, engine and transmission to get the car going in the morning. And the meditation quiets my mind, centers me, and improves my judgment. You probably have your own tricks for raising your spirits. Now is the time to use them.

One of my good friends wakes up each morning by listing the things she has to be grateful for. She thanks God, or life, or whatever you will, for the good things that surround her and nurture her. It is a wonderful practice, and she is known for her sunny disposition throughout the rest of the day.

The Hawaiians have a good tradition in this area. Whenever there is a situation of chronic resentment, anger or disagreement in the family or the community, they undertake a process called ho'oponopono. All involved sit down to discuss the matter, going into it deeply, working hard, until understanding and resolution is reached. Quakers have a similar process, called a "threshing session". The result is spiritual healing. I recommend this strongly for cancer patients. If you have an unsettled quarrel with a sibling, parent, child or colleague, get it out, settle it, get rid of it. For it is needlessly robbing you of energy. Forgiveness and gratitude are both energy-preservers. If you make a habit of them, you will notice the difference.

Occasionally, during my surgical practice, the question of prayer would arise. If requested, I would pray for or with a patient, but I never made it a habit. I think both I and the patient felt that, if his surgeon was praying for him, then he must really be in bad shape! But this is a superficial way to look at it.

In his book *Healing Words*, Larry Dossey deals with prayer and medicine. It is a good discussion of the question, and I recommend it. As a sceptic, Dr. Dossey started out trying to disprove the usefulness of prayer, studying extensively the evidence for its effectiveness. To his surprise and chagrin, he found that there is an increasing body of statistically significant proof that prayer is a therapeutic help. He concluded by feeling that, as a physician, withholding prayer from his patients is as remiss as failing to use a recently proven drug.

Dossey says he has no idea how or why it works—it is a mystery into which we have no knowledge—perhaps similar to the mystery regarding the existence of God. In other words, it is a matter of faith. Yet it can be a source of positive energy, if you will. We don't really know where it comes from, but we can feel its healing power if we are sensitive to it. It seems to me that prayers of hope and gratitude are a little bit like the learned optimism of Seligman, in religious rather than psychological terms—you believe something good is going to happen, and it usually does.

Visualization can play a role here. Carl Simonton et al. describe the process in their classic book *Getting Well Again*. Dr. Simonton shows the usefulness of positive mental images in dealing with cancer. Patients are trained to visualize their white blood cells as attacking and destroying cancer cells. He stresses how we should see the immune system as being more potent than the cancer cells, and there is good evidence for the truth of this. Dr. Simonton, a radiation oncologist, states that "…while we in cancer therapy appreciate that medicine can do a great deal, we believe that the body's basic defenses eliminating the cancerous cells is the essential aspect in regaining health."

Visualization is, really, not a new or "far-out" idea—we do it all the time, both positively and negatively, though we may not realize what we are doing. When we "see" a coming event in our mind's eye, expecting it to be pleasurable and comfortable, it usually is— like dinner out with friends at a favorite restaurant. On the other hand, a dreaded confrontation with an adversary is usually just as unpleasant as we expect it to be. And we program our nervous system (and our immune system as well, it turns out) to react according to our predictions. But if you anticipate goodness, you become a "swimmer of the deep," expecting to reach a far-off point, stroking strongly and confidently, and you reach your goal.

A CURE FOR CANCER

We make no claim of having found the cure for cancer. As noted above, uncounted numbers of patients have discovered their own cures, surviving when everyone around them had given them up for lost, with or without the help of conventional medical measures. We think it increasingly apparent that what makes the difference for these fortunate ones is that they find something or somethings to "jump-start" a protective complex that had been failing them. What we have described is the way the thing works, the causality of cancer. We think we've made sense of what has been a great riddle.

Finding your own personal cure is now up to you. No one else knows what is likely to heal you and what will probably not. Physicians are instructors and guides, their instruments and drugs only aides. When I operate on a patient, I rearrange his or her anatomy, but a force far stronger and more skillful than I knits tissues together to make them whole. This is a time to take stock of yourself and discover what is best for you. Although made from the same tissues, we are all different—physically, emotionally, even biochemically. Recent studies have shown that some people thrive on vegetarian diets, others need some red meat. "One man's meat is another man's poison," has a lot of truth to it. Find out what nourishes you, in every sense of the term.

Your illness is a wake up call, time to make your health a priority. We will suggest a menu of things to look into: immune system stimulants (supplements and nutrients), spiritual resources, meditation, and exercise, to name a few. Consider your energy stores. Norman Cousins made a strong case for the healing power of laughter. Heal your relationships, increase fellowship—perhaps in cancer support groups. Use music, art and entertainment. Andrew Weil has an excellent compact disc incorporating music and meditation called, "Sound Body, Sound Mind."

There is another analogy that comes to mind. I have a 20 year old four cylinder car that won't make it over a long hill if one of the cylinders is misfiring. And I think it is the same with cancer therapy. We need all four "cylinders"—tumor destruction, an intact immune system, adequate energy, and a will to live—to get us up the hill.

So I wish to wake up your mind to what your body needs and to what empowers you spiritually. Your mind can then choose, from this feast of options we have presented, what suits you best. Once yoking together mind, body and spirit, you will be well on your way to healing.

3

Recent Developments in Cancer Treatment

Ian Okazaki, M.D.
Hawai'i Pacific Health
Straub Medical Center
Division of Hematology/Oncology
Honolulu, Hawaii

I. Introduction

About one in eight people in the United States will be afflicted by cancer in their lifetime. The development of cancer is a multifactorial process resulting from the interaction of environmental and genetic factors. Research has uncovered some of the environmental factors that contribute to carcinogenesis such as viruses, inflammation, toxins, radiation, and diet. Certain viruses have been associated with initiation and proliferation of cancer cells (1). The Epstein Barr virus is associated with nasopharyngeal carcinoma and Burkitt's lymphoma, the human papilloma virus with cervical cancer, while the human herpes virus 8 has been shown to be associated with development of Kaposi's sarcoma. High-fat diet has been associated with an increased risk of breast, colon, kidney and other cancers. Exposure to toxins or radiation, as well as chronic infection or inflammation has also been linked to cancer formation. There are numerous acquired genetic mutations in addition to

23

amplified function of normal genes that initiate or contribute to cancer propagation (2). Mutations in the BRCA1 and BRCA2 genes are directly associated with breast cancer as well as ovarian cancer formation. Mutations or increased expression of molecular switches within the cell including membrane receptors such as c-kit and epidermal growth factor receptor, and intracellular molecules such as ras and raf, are detected in many cancers consistent with their role in proliferation of cancer cells. Tumor suppressor genes p53, retinoblastoma gene, and PTEN, regulate critical pathways in cell metabolism and cell division. Typically, the loss of one copy (allele) of the tumor suppressor gene and mutation of the remaining allele leads to loss of tumor suppressor function resulting in uninhibited cell growth and proliferation. Cancer cells are known to undergo a series of mutational events that initiate the malignant process and lead to a more aggressive cancer that spreads or metastasizes and acquires drug resistance. Understanding the various mutational events in the process of cancer progression is critical for the development of new cancer therapies.

The treatment of cancer usually relies on multimodality treatment including surgery, radiation therapy, chemotherapy (3), targeted therapy, and immunotherapy. Surgery is often the mainstay of cancer treatment since it allows complete removal of the tumor at its site of origin. Although cancer cells may not be evident at the surgical margins, the ability of cancers to invade tissues and lymphatic and vascular channels increases the risk of local recurrence as well as dissemination to distant sites (metastasis) despite surgery. Radiation therapy reduces the risk of local tumor recurrence by treating the surrounding tissues with ionizing radiation that directly kills residual cancer cells. Chemotherapy, targeted therapy, and immunotherapy, on the other hand, are systemic treatments that target cancer cells at their origins as well as those cells that may have traveled to distant sites. Several of the mutations affecting cell metabolism, uncovered by recent advances in cancer research, have led to development of novel agents capable of selectively targeting cancer cells carrying these mutations. In recent years, the search for more effective combination chemotherapy regimens and the incorporation of new drugs in the fight against cancer have accelerated considerably due to laboratory research and patient participation in clinical trials. The results of these developments have improved the response to therapy leading to extended patient survival and enhanced quality of life.

II. Surgery

Surgery is critical in the diagnosis and treatment of cancer. Surgical procedures can be diagnostic, therapeutic, or palliative. Diagnostic surgery consists of removal of the tumor or biopsy of a portion of the tumor to establish a diagnosis. Surgery is sometimes required to determine the stage or extent of involvement of the cancer. Surgery is curative for many early stage cancers. Lung, colon, prostate, kidney, bladder, head and neck and most skin cancers have an excellent prognosis if surgery is performed in the earliest stages. Breast cancer surgery is unique in that radiation therapy is often administered after removal of the primary tumor (lumpectomy), in order to help prevent local recurrence. In some instances, particularly for those patients with a genetic predisposition to cancer, prophylactic surgery is performed to remove tissues or organs at high risk for cancer development such as breast, ovarian and colon cancer (4).

For those cancers treated with surgery alone, the risk of recurrence depends on size and grade of the tumor, the extent of lymphatic or vascular invasion, and spread of tumor to regional lymph nodes among other pathologic features. Tumors at higher risk of recurrence and metastasis are often treated with radiation therapy and or chemotherapy administered before (neoadjuvant) or after (adjuvant) surgery. The appropriate treatment is usually individualized for each patient and involves consultation with a team of cancer specialists that includes members of the surgery, pathology, medical oncology, radiation oncology, and nursing. Recent developments in cancer surgery include minimally invasive techniques in which fiberoptic devices are used for video-assisted tumor resection, as well as radiofrequency ablation, cryotherapy, and photocoagulation therapy of tumors (5). As with other surgical procedures, a second opinion is often beneficial particularly for those cancers that are unusual or occur rarely.

Surgery is not utilized solely for early stage cancer. For example, resection of a solitary metastasis has a beneficial effect on survival for many cancer types even though the cancer has spread beyond its site of origin. Surgery is sometimes required to prevent or treat complications associated with advanced cancer. Such palliative surgical procedures are performed to relieve bowel or urinary tract obstruction, to alleviate pain or pressure associated with a rapidly growing mass, or to stop bleeding. A skilled surgeon is, therefore, a key member of the cancer care team who is often involved at all stages of cancer treatment.

III. Radiation Therapy

Radiation therapy utilizes ionizing radiation that disrupts and kills proliferating cancer cells. There are different mechanisms for delivery of radiation therapy including external beam radiation, insertion of radioactive implants into the tumor called brachytherapy, and injection of radioactive isotopes or radionuclides. Radiation therapy is curative for several cancer types such as early stage Hodgkin's and non-Hodgkin's lymphoma, prostate cancer, thyroid cancer, certain brain tumors, and seminoma, among others. Adjuvant radiation therapy can be utilized after surgery to treat the area surrounding the primary cancer to prevent local recurrence as in breast, prostate, gastric, and head and neck cancer, and some sarcomas. In this setting, radiation can improve cure rates compared with surgery alone. Alternatively, radiation may be used instead of surgery particularly if surgery is not feasible because of location or extent of the cancer.

Certain cancers are treated with concurrent administration of chemotherapy and radiation therapy, which is more effective than either therapy alone. Localized anal cancer can be cured by concurrent chemotherapy and radiation therapy. Lung cancer that has spread to lymph nodes in the chest (stage III) is usually not amenable to surgery, but 10-20% of patients achieve long-term remission following concurrent chemoradiation. Further, laryngeal cancer treated with chemoradiation is as effective as surgery and allows preservation of the larynx and vocal cord function. In some instances, such as head and neck, esophagus, gastric, bladder cancer, and rectal cancer, neoadjuvant chemoradiation therapy (before surgery) helps to shrink the tumor and potentially treats microscopic metastases prior to definitive surgery. The positive outcomes of chemoradiation on these and other types of cancer has led to further research to optimize chemoradiation as compared to surgery or radiation alone.

As with surgery, radiation therapy also provides symptom relief for advanced cancers. Pain caused by invasive cancer in the primary or metastatic sites is effectively alleviated by radiation. Radiation is utilized to treat progressive tumor growth in any site such as the brain, abdomen, pelvis, soft tissues, or bone, and is also used to treat or prevent obstruction in critical areas such as the lung, esophagus, and abdomen. Further, bleeding from tumors can be managed successfully with radiation therapy.

For external beam radiation, a CT scan is used to determine the precise area to be treated. A linear accelerator is programmed to deliver radiation directly to the tumor with minimal exposure to the surrounding tissues. Radiation is delivered in small doses or fractions on a daily or sometimes twice daily basis until the desired cumulative dose is reached. The total radiation dose is determined by the type of cancer being treated and the organ in which it arises. General side effects of radiation include fatigue, malaise, and nausea, but specific effects depend on the site of radiation treatment and the cumulative dose used. For example, treatment of head and neck cancer is often associated with mouth sores and sore throat. Esophageal cancer treatment causes chest pain, cough, and difficulty swallowing.

Advances in technology have improved radiation treatment (6) such as intensity-modulated radiation therapy (IMRT), which allows more precise dosing of the tumor with minimal exposure of surrounding tissues. Brachytherapy involves implantation of radioactive seeds or needles directly into tumor tissues in order to deliver high doses of radiation. Brachytherapy has been especially successful in the treatment of prostate cancer. New techniques in radiation therapy have certainly expanded the effective treatment alternatives for some cancers.

IV. Chemotherapy

The first class of chemotherapy drugs used clinically to treat cancer was the alkylating agents that had their origins as nerve gas (mustard gas) developed by the military. At about the same time, antimetabolites that function as antifolate agents were noted to have a beneficial effect in the treatment of childhood leukemia. There are now many different classes of chemotherapy agents that have specific effects on different aspects of cell metabolism (7). A partial list of the different classes of chemotherapy drugs is listed in Table I. The alkylating agents such as cyclophosphamide, nitrogen mustard, and chlorambucil inhibit cell division by binding to, or cross-linking DNA strands. The platinum containing compounds, cisplatin, carboplatin, oxaliplatin, alter the DNA strands, which prevents replication and transcription of DNA critical to cell function. Antimetabolites such as methotrexate, 5-fluorouracil, 6-mercaptopurine, cytosine arabinoside, and gemcitabine inhibit nucleic acid synthesis thereby affecting DNA and RNA metabolism. The topoisomerase inhibitors, such as the camptothecins (topotecan, irinotecan), epipodophyllotoxins (etoposide), and anthracyclines (doxorubicin, mitoxantrone) prevent repair of DNA strand breaks, which leads to cell death or apoptosis. The antimicrotubule agents include the vinca alkaloids (vincristine, vinorelbine), taxanes (paclitaxel, docetaxel), and estramustine, which interact with tubulin and inhibit microtubule function that disrupts the mitotic (cell division) process as well as non-mitotic functions of microtubules. There are several chemotherapy agents that have unique mechanisms of action. For example, DNA methylation and histone deacetylation are potential targets for chemotherapy drugs. Cancer-promoting genes called oncogenes may initiate and accelerate tumor formation by enhancing DNA methylation and histone deacetylation, which suppresses normal gene function including those essential for controlling cell growth. 5-azacitidine induces DNA demethylation and has modest activity in diseases of the bone marrow called myelodysplastic syndromes. Bortezomib, carfilzomib, and ixazomib are novel histone deacetylase inhibitors that are quite active in multiple myeloma.

There is often an additive or synergistic activity when chemotherapy agents are used in combination. Combination chemotherapy interferes with proliferation and spread of cancer cells by altering DNA function and cellular metabolism at critical sites. The drug combinations tend to be non-cross-resistant so that cancer cells are attacked by agents having different mechanisms of action. Chemotherapy is administered repeatedly and should be delivered as frequently as possible to optimize tumor exposure to the drugs and enhance incremental tumor cell kill (8). High doses of chemotherapy may overcome drug resistance, but patients often need autologous blood stem cell transplantation to rescue the bone marrow from the toxic effects of chemotherapy. High-dose chemotherapy followed by autologous peripheral blood stem cell transplantation has become useful in the treatment of multiple myeloma, and some forms of lymphoma (9).

Chemotherapy is curative for some types of lymphoma and leukemia, and testicular cancer. For all other types of cancer, combined modality treatment utilizing surgery, radiation therapy, and chemotherapy often provides superior results compared with that of each modality alone. Neoadjuvant chemotherapy is used prior to definitive surgery in order to shrink the tumor and allow a less mutilating surgery. Neoadjuvant chemotherapy has proven effective for breast, head and neck, esophagus, gastric, rectal, and bladder cancer, and some sarcomas. Adjuvant chemotherapy administered after primary treatment is effective in reducing the risk of recurrence after surgery for most tumor types including breast, lung, gastric, colorectal, pancreas, urothelial, and ovarian, cancer. In advanced stages of cancer, chemotherapy is commonly used to provide relief from cancer-related symptoms. In this setting, the side effects of chemotherapy must be balanced against its potential benefits. Even with metastatic cancer that is not curable, chemotherapy can improve the overall survival for those patients with lung, colon, breast, and other cancer types, compared with observation alone. New drug discovery and cancer clinical trials are essential in order to achieve significant improvement in cancer treatment outcomes.

The side effects of chemotherapy are varied and depend, in part, on the drug being used. Chemotherapy will affect normal cells that divide regularly such as those in the skin, including hair follicles and nails, intestines and bone marrow. The effects on normal cells and tissues are responsible for some of the chemotherapy-induced side effects. Most chemotherapy drugs are associated with fatigue, malaise, anorexia, weight loss, mouth sores, nausea, vomiting, diarrhea or constipation, and suppression of blood cell production. Hair loss is a consequence of some, but not all, chemotherapy agents. The effects of chemotherapy on the bone marrow leads to the lowering of the blood cell counts that results in anemia and an increased the risk of infection and bleeding. Routine administration of blood and bone marrow growth factors helps speed recovery of blood cell counts in between treatments and allows chemotherapy to be administered on schedule and at full doses. Anticipation of side effects and proper management of chemotherapy-induced symptoms is as important as the chemotherapy regimen selected for cancer treatment.

V. Hormonal Therapy.

Hormonal treatments are effective in cancers that are driven by hormones such as breast, prostate and endometrial cancer. The aromatase inhibitors anastrozole, letrozole and exemestane are drugs that inhibit estrogen synthesis and are used to treat hormone receptor-positive breast cancer. In fact, the aromatase inhibitors demonstrated superior activity compared to tamoxifen in the treatment of breast cancer in the postmenopausal population (10). Similarly, newer agents for the treatment of prostate cancer enhance testosterone depletion especially in the sites of metastases, which helps to improve progression-free survival and successfully delays the onset of prostate cancer-related complications.

VI. Targeted Therapies.

Intensive research in recent years has resulted in the development of numerous new anticancer agents that target specific cell receptors and intracellular switches that are responsible, in part, for controlling cell growth and cancer formation. Some of these drugs have proven effective in the treatment of several types of cancer (11). In addition, the side effect profiles of these drugs are quite different than that of standard chemotherapy. The development of imatinib was revolutionary as the first drug of its kind to specifically inhibit the mutated BCR-ABL tyrosine kinase enzyme present in chronic myelogenous leukemia (CML) resulting in remission and potential cure of the disease. CML is characterized by a unique rearrangement between chromosome 9 and chromosome 22. This DNA rearrangement generates the abnormal BCR-ABL kinase, which permits uncontrolled cell growth. Previously, the only curative therapy for CML had been allogeneic bone marrow transplantation and imatinib offers an effective treatment particularly for older patients and those patients not eligible for the transplantation procedure. Imatinib also inhibits the mutated and overactive cell membrane receptor kinase called c-kit that is present in gastrointestinal stromal tumors (abdominal sarcoma).

Erlotinib, gefitinib, and osimertinib are agents that inhibit the epidermal growth factor receptor (EGFR) kinase activity and are being used in the treatment of advanced lung cancer harboring specific EGFR mutations (12).

Sorafenib inhibits RAF kinase, vascular endothelial growth factor receptor (VEGFR), and platelet-derived growth factor receptor (PDGFR), which are three different switches controlling cancer cell proliferation. Sorafenib is one of the first multi-tyrosine kinase inhibitors that is used to treat metastatic liver, kidney, thyroid cancers and desmoid tumors (13). Sunitinib is another multi-tyrosine kinase inhibitor that targets VEGFR and PDGFR involved in oncogenesis and tumor cell proliferation. It is used to treat gastrointestinal stromal tumors, pancreatic neuroendocrine tumors, kidney cancer, leukemias, and other solid tumors (14). There are numerous other targeted therapies that are proven effective in the treatment of malignancies that possess favorable or activating mutations amenable to mutation-specific inhibitors. There is ongoing research testing targeted therapies against cancers of all types that possess mutations known to be susceptible to these agents regardless of primary site of malignancy.

VII. Immunotherapy.

Biologic therapy including cytokines, therapeutic monoclonal antibodies, and cell-mediated immunity, exert their effects by stimulating immune function to enhance host defense against cancer cells. One of the earliest forms of immunotherapy consisted of the nonspecific activation of immune cells to prevent cancer recurrence or control cancer cell progression. Urologists used bacille Calmette-Guérin (BCG) a mycobacterium protein that is instilled into the bladder to activate local immune cells since the 1930s, in order to prevent recurrence of bladder cancer in situ and non-muscle invasive bladder cancer. FDA approval for BCG as intravesicular therapy for non-muscle invasive bladder cancer was granted in 1990.

Cytokines. Cytokines are biologic proteins that boost immune function (15). Interferon is a cytokine that affects cell cycle regulation, promotes unveiling of tumor cells so that they are recognized by normal immune surveillance, and directly activates immune function. Interferons have beneficial effects in melanoma, renal cell carcinoma and Kaposi's sarcoma. The cytokine interleukin-2 induces expression of other immune-stimulating cytokines and activates the tumor-fighting immune cells including T lymphocytes and natural killer (NK) cells. IL-2 therapy has modest activity against advanced melanoma and renal cell carcinoma but has significant treatment-associated toxicity. IL-2 was approved for use in the treatment of metastatic renal cell carcinoma in 1992, and for metastatic melanoma in 1998.

Monoclonal Antibodies. Monoclonal antibodies have been generated that target proteins responsible for stimulating cell growth (growth factors) and the molecules on the cell surface that bind to these growth factors (growth factor receptors) that function to modulate cell function and proliferation. Trastuzumab is one such antibody directed against the HER2/neu (erbB2) receptor that is expressed on up to 25% of breast cancers (16, 17). Chemotherapy and trastuzumab combinations provide superior response rates and survival compared with chemotherapy alone in the treatment of metastatic HER2/neu-positive breast cancer. Further, data from clinical trials established the role of chemotherapy and trastuzumab administered after surgery, which significantly reduced the risk of cancer recurrence and mortality in early stage HER2/neu-positive breast cancer. There are trastuzumab-chemotherapy conjugates such as ado-trastuzumab emtansine consisting of a HER2-targeted antibody conjugated with a microtubule inhibitor that was approved February 22, 2013, for late stage HER2/neu-positive breast cancer, and as adjuvant therapy for early stage HER2/neu-positive breast cancer in May 3, 2019.

Another monoclonal antibody bevacizumab binds vascular endothelial growth factor (VEGF) and inhibits blood vessel formation (angiogenesis), essential for tumor growth (18). The use of bevacizumab with or without chemotherapy is proven effective in the treatment of metastatic colon, lung, ovarian, and brain cancers and was approved for medical use in 2004.

Rituximab is a monoclonal antibody directed against CD20 that is expressed on B-cell non-Hodgkin's lymphomas (19). Rituximab in combination with chemotherapy has significantly improved outcomes in lymphoma therapy. The monoclonal antibody cetuximab, targets the epidermal growth factor receptor that is present at high levels in several malignancies (20). This monoclonal antibody is being used clinically in the treatment of metastatic colon cancer and squamous cell carcinoma of the head and neck. Radioimmunoconjugates are monoclonal antibodies attached to radioactive agents that bind to a specific tumor cell protein allowing the toxic effects of radiation to penetrate the tumor mass (21). Radioimmunoconjugates such as tositumomab (^{131}I-anti-CD20 monoclonal antibody) and ibritumomab (^{90}Y-anti-CD20 monoclonal antibody) are effective in inducing remissions in relapsed follicular non-Hodgkin's lymphoma. Identification of other molecules specifically expressed on tumor cells will help to create other monoclonal antibodies that specifically bind to these molecules to effect antitumor responses.

Checkpoint Inhibitors. Immune checkpoint inhibition has been a revolutionary breakthrough in the treatment of cancer

(22). Ipilimumab, a monoclonal antibody that blocks the immune checkpoint molecule CTLA-4 on the T-cell, was the first such agent approved in 2011 for the treatment of advanced melanoma. Other checkpoint inhibitor monoclonal antibodies bind to and block function of PD-1 on T-cells or PD-L1 on tumor cells and other cells in the peripheral tissues. Checkpoint inhibition occurs when PD-L1 on tumor cells bind to PD-1 on T cells, or B7-1/B7-2 on antigen presenting cells (APC) bind to CTLA-4 on T-cells to hold immune responses in check and avoids excessive or inappropriate T-cell responses. Blocking the binding of PD-1 to PD-L1 or B7-1/B7-2 to CTLA-4, on the other hand, allows T-cells to remain in an activated state and sustain tumor target killing, and circumvents the innate negative regulation that shuts off T-cell killing. Checkpoint inhibition therapy has demonstrated anti-tumor activity against a rather broad range of tumor types including head and neck, lung, liver, gastric, esophageal, kidney, urothelial, cervical, and skin (melanoma, Merkel cell, squamous cell) cancers, and some forms of Hodgkin lymphoma, non-Hodgkin lymphoma, "triple-negative" breast cancer, and colorectal cancer, and any mismatch repair-deficient solid tumors. Examples of checkpoint inhibitor therapies include the anti-CTLA-4 monoclonal antibody ipilimumab, anti-PD-1 monoclonal antibodies cemiplimab, nivolumab, and pembrolizumab, and anti-PD-L1 monoclonal antibodies atezolizumab, avelumab, durvalumab. Checkpoint inhibitor therapy is associated with a broad array of immune-related adverse events due to activation of immune cells in tissues and organs not necessarily associated with sites of tumor or metastases. These immune-related adverse events can mimic autoimmune conditions and might require steroids (prednisone or methylprednisolone) to reverse the brisk immune response (23).

Cell-mediated Immune Therapy. Cell-mediated immune therapy such as vaccines and adoptive immune therapy (immune cell infusions) have limited application but continues to be an active area of research. Vaccines function to enhance recognition of unique tumor proteins by cytotoxic T lymphocytes (CTL) or killer T cells that become activated by the vaccine and kill cancer cells possessing the tumor-specific proteins (24). Vaccines have demonstrated modest responses in melanoma and renal cell carcinoma. Sipuleucel T is one such vaccine that was FDA-approved April 29, 2010 (25), for the treatment of castrate-resistant prostate cancer. On the other hand, vaccines that generate an immune response against human papilloma virus have proven effective in the prevention of cervical cancer.

Adoptive immune therapy consists of isolation and proliferation of a population of immune cells in the laboratory and subsequent infusion of these cells back into the patient so that the expanded army of CTL target and kill cancer cells (26). Adoptive immune therapy had its origins in allogeneic bone marrow transplantation dating back to 1956, and has become curative therapy for relapsed and refractory leukemia and lymphoma. Chimeric Antigen Receptor-expressing T-cells (CAR T-cell) therapy is a rapidly developing field in cancer therapy and involves isolation of T-cells from the patient's blood, insertion of a gene that produces a special receptor on the T cell surface that recognizes and binds to a specific protein on the patient's cancer cells. The genetically engineered CAR T-cell population is expanded to the millions in the laboratory before they are infused back into the patient. This form of adoptive immunotherapy, or T cell transfer, is FDA-approved for the treatment of children and adolescents with relapsed and refractory acute lymphoblastic leukemia (27), and for relapsed and refractory diffuse large B cell non-Hodgkin lymphoma (28). CAR T-cells specifically target the malignant cell population, but can also have serious side effects related to the release of cytokines or immune molecules, in particular interleukin-6 (IL-6), that stimulates and enhances the immune response leading to high fevers, large drops in blood pressure, depletion of normal B-cells, seizures, and cerebral edema. These serious side effects, called cytokine release syndrome, are now more easily recognized and managed (29). Improvements in CAR T-cell therapy is associated with better, more durable outcomes for leukemia and lymphoma. CAR T-cell or other adoptive cell-mediated immune therapies are being tested against solid tumors including melanoma, cervical cancer, and sarcoma.

VIII. Coordination of Care.

The medical oncologist and oncology nursing staff are responsible for leading the patient through the process required for diagnosis and staging of the cancer and making the appropriate referrals for surgery and radiation oncology consultation. Patients with cancer also require the services of the pharmacist, dietician, social worker, and spiritual ministries, and the medical oncology staff should be responsible for the coordination of care that is needed for each patient. Patients should expect frequent visits to the medical oncologist since treatment requires close monitoring for management of side effects and frequent assessment of response to treatment. The successful navigation through the course of cancer care from diagnosis through treatment requires the integration of the evidence-based medical decision making and interventions with the innate emotional and spiritual component of healing. Patients and care-givers often seek emotional and spiritual counsel outside of the confines of traditional medical practice. It is essential for the oncology team to be able to address the palliative and symptom-based care along with the spiritual issues of each patient throughout the course of cancer care.

IX. Clinical Trials

A cancer clinical trial is a research study using human subjects to find better ways for prevention, diagnosis and treatment of cancer. Over 1.7 million cancer cases were diagnosed in 2019 and cancer is the second leading cause of death after cardiac disease. It may take up to 10-15 years from the time of discovery of a drug to its approval for use in patients, and clinical trials play an important role in the development of effective cancer treatments. A phase I clinical trial establishes drug safety and finds the appropriate dose to be used for disease treatment. A phase II study further evaluates drug safety and is designed to demonstrate efficacy of the drug against a specific cancer type. Subsequent phase III clinical trials compare the experimental drug, or drug combination against the current standard therapy. Clinical trials are invaluable in advancing new cancer treatments and an appropriate trial should be considered for all patients diagnosed with cancer. Unfortunately, fewer than 5% of adults participate in cancer clinical trials, and large academic centers often enroll only 15% of their patients into cancer clinical trials (30). This rate of clinical trial participation certainly slows the progress of cancer research. Patients should be assured of the scientific merit of the study and must be made aware of the fact that they are protected by Research Subjects' Protection Programs available at all participating cancer treatment facilities. There are several benefits of clinical trial participation including the fact that research subjects are assured comprehensive medical care and close follow-up. A clinical trial often provides access to new drugs or devices that are not available outside of the experimental protocol, particularly when no good treatment alternatives are available. Superior patient outcomes are often observed when a patient takes an active role in his or her own care that is afforded by clinical trial participation. Lastly clinical trials serve to advance cancer care that will benefit others with cancer in the future. The patient's cancer team as well as relatives and caregivers remain instrumental in encouraging clinical trial participation in effort to expand each patient's treatment options and improve quality of life.

References

1. Butel JS. Viral carcinogenesis: revelation of molecular mechanisms and etiology of human disease. Carcinogenesis. 2000, 21:405-26.

2. Ajani J, Algood V. Molecular mechanisms in cancer: what should clinicians know?
Semin Oncol. 2005, 32(6 Suppl 8):2-4.

3. Boyle FM, Robinson E, Dunn SM, Heinrich PC. Multidisciplinary care in cancer: the fellowship of the ring. J Clin Oncol. 2005, 23:916-20.

4. Bertagnolli MM. Surgical prevention of cancer. J Clin Oncol. 2005, 23:324-32.

5. Coldwell DM, Sewell PE. The expanding role of interventional radiology in the supportive care of the oncology patient: from diagnosis to therapy. Semin Oncol. 2005 32:169-73.

6. Elshaikh M, Ljungman M, Ten Haken R, Lichter AS. Advances in Radiation Oncology. Annu Rev Med. 2005, Oct 19

7. Connors T. Anticancer Drug Development: The Way Forward. Oncologist. 1996, 1:180-181.

8. Hudis CA, Schmitz N. Dose-dense chemotherapy in breast cancer and lymphoma. Semin Oncol. 2004, 31(3 Suppl 8):19-26.

9. Craddock C. Haemopoietic stem-cell transplantation: recent progress and future promise. Lancet Oncol. 2000, 1:227-34.

10. Stasser-Weippl K, Goss PE. Advances in adjuvant hormonal therapy for postmenopausal women. J Clin Oncol. 2005, 23:1751-9.

11. Smith JK, Mamoon NM, Duhe RJ. Emerging roles of targeted small molecule protein-tyrosine kinase inhibitors in cancer therapy. Oncol Res. 2004, 14:175-225.

12. EGFR-targeted therapy. Loredana Vecchione, Bart Jacobs, Nicola Normanno, Fortunato Ciardiello, Sabine Tejpar. Experimental Cell Research. 15 November 2011, Volume 317(19): 2765-2771

13. Escudier B, Eisen T, Stadler WM, et al; for TARGET Study Group. Sorafenib in advanced clear-cell renal-cell carcinoma. N Engl J Med. 2007; 356(2):125-134.

14. Understanding the molecular-based mechanism of action of the tyrosine kinase inhibitor: sunitinib. Carrato Mena, Alfredo; Grande Pulido, Enrique; Guillén-Ponce, Carmen. Anti-Cancer Drugs: January 2010, Volume 21:S3-S11.

15. Tagawa M. Cytokine therapy for cancer. Curr Pharm Des. 2000, 6:681-99.

16. Hortobagyi GN. Overview of treatment results with trastuzumab (Herceptin) in metastatic breast cancer. Semin Oncol. 2001, 28(6 Suppl 18):43-7.

17. Piccart-Gebhart MJ, Procter M, Leyland-Jones B, Goldhirsch A, Untch M, Smith I, Gianni L, Baselga J, Bell R, Jackisch C, Cameron D, Dowsett M, Barrios CH, Steger G, Huang CS, Andersson M, Inbar M, Lichinister M, Lnag I, Nitz U, Iwata H, Thomssen C, Lohrisch C, Suter TM, Ruschoff J, Suto T, Greatorex V, Ward C, Straehle C, McFadden E, Dolci MS, Gelber RD; Herceptin Adjuvant (HERA) Trial Study Team. Trastuzumab after adjuvant chemotherapy in HER2-positive breast cancer. N Engl J Med. 2005, 353:1659-72.

18. Zondor SD, Medina PJ. Bevacizumab: an angiogenesis inhibitor with efficacy in colorectal and other malignancies. Ann Pharmacother. 2004, 38:1258-64.

19. Plosker GL, Figitt DP. Rituximab: a review of its use in non-Hodgkin's lymphoma and chronic lymphocytic leukaemia. Drugs. 2003, 63:803-43.

20. El-Rayes BF, LoRusso PM. Targeting the epidermal growth factor receptor. Br J Cancer. 2004, 91:418-24.

21. Goldenberg DM. The role of radiolabeled antibodies in the treatment of non-Hodgkin's lymphoma: the coming of age of radioimmunotherapy. Crit Rev Oncol Hematol. 2001, 39:195-201.

22. Immune Checkpoint Blockade in Cancer Therapy. Michael A. Postow, Margaret K. Callahan, and Jedd D. Wolchok. J Clin Oncol. 2015 Jun 10; 33(17): 1974–1982.

23. Management of Immune-Related Adverse Events in Patients Treated With Immune Checkpoint Inhibitor Therapy: American Society of Clinical Oncology Clinical Practice Guideline. Julie R. Brahmer, Christina Lacchetti, Bryan J. Schneider, Michael B. Atkins, Kelly J. Brassil, Jeffrey M. Caterino, Ian Chau, Marc S. Ernstoff, Jennifer M. Gardner, Pamela Ginex, Sigrun

Hallmeyer, Jennifer Holter Chakrabarty, Natasha B. Leighl, Jennifer S. Mammen, David F. McDermott, Aung Naing, Loretta J. Nastoupil, Tanyanika Phillips, Laura D. Porter, Igor Puzanov, Cristina A. Reichner, Bianca D. Santomasso, Carole Seigel, Alexander Spira, Maria E. Suarez-Almazor, Yinghong Wang, MD, Jeffrey S. Weber, Jedd D. Wolchok, and John A. Thompson, collaboration with the National Comprehensive Cancer Network. J Clin Oncol. 2018 Jun 10; 36(17): 1714–1768.

24. Bonnefoy JY. Cancer vaccines. Expert Opin Ther Targets. 2004, 8:521-5.

25. Sipuleucel-T immunotherapy for castration-resistant prostate cancer. Kantoff PW; Higano CS; Shore ND; Berger ER; Small EJ; Penson DF; Redfern CH; Ferrari AC; Dreicer R; Sims RB; Xu Y; Frohlich MW; Schellhammer PF (July 2010). N. Engl. J. Med. 363 (5): 411–22.

26. Hillman GG, Haas GP, Wahl WH, Callewaert DM. Adoptive immunotherapy of cancer: biological response modifiers and cytotoxic cell therapy. Biotherapy. 1992, 5:119-29.

27. Efficacy and Toxicity Management of 19-28z CAR T Cell Therapy in B Cell Acute Lymphoblastic Leukemia. Marco L. Davila[1], Isabelle Riviere, Xiuyan Wang[4], et al. Science Translational Medicine, 19 Feb 2014: Vol. 6, Issue 224, pp. 224ra25

28. Axicabtagene Ciloleucel CAR T-Cell Therapy in Refractory Large B-Cell Lymphoma. Neelapu SS, Locke FL, Bartlett NL, Lekakis LJ, Miklos DB, Jacobson CA, Braunschweig I, Oluwole OO, Siddiqi T, Lin Y, Timmerman JM, Stiff PJ, Friedberg JW[1], Flinn IW, Goy A, Hill BT, Smith MR, Deol A, Farooq U, McSweeney P, Munoz J, Avivi I, Castro JE, Westin JR, Chavez JC, Ghobadi A, Komanduri KV, Levy R, Jacobsen ED, Witzig TE, Reagan P, Bot A, Rossi J, Navale L, Jiang Y, Aycock J, Elias M, Chang D[1], Wiezorek J, Go WY. N Engl J Med. 2017 Dec 28; 377(26):2531-2544. doi: 10. 1056/NEJMoa1707447. Epub 2017 Dec 10.

29. Toxicity and management in CAR T-cell therapy. Challice L Bonifant, Hollie J Jackson, Renier J Brentjens, Kevin J Curran. Molecular Therapy Oncolytics Volume 3, 2016, 16011.

30. Tournoux C, Katsahian S, Chevret S, Levy V. Factors influencing inclusion of patients with malignancies in clinical trials. Cancer. 2005, 106:258-270.

Table 1. Classes of chemotherapeutic agents.

Class	Mechanism of action	Examples
Alkylating agents	Binds and cross links DNA and prevents cell division.	Cyclophosphamide: breast cancer, lymphoma. Chlorambucil: chronic lymphocytic leukemia. Nitrogen mustard: Hodgkin's lymphoma.
Platinum-containing	Interstrand and intrastrand cross linking of DNA, which prevents replication and transcription of DNA.	Cisplatin: lung, bladder cancer, germ cell tumors. Carboplatin: lung, ovarian cancer. Oxaliplatin: colon cancer.
Antimetabolites	Inhibits nucleic acid synthesis, which affects DNA and RNA metabolism.	Methotrexate: breast, bladder cancer, lymphoma. 5-fluorouracil: gastric, colon cancer. Gemcitabine: lung, breast, pancreas, bladder cancer.
Topoisomerase inhibitors	Prevents repair of DNA strand breaks, which leads to cell death or apoptosis.	Irinotecan: colon, gastric cancer. Etoposide: lung cancer, lymphoma, leukemia. Doxorubicin: breast cancer, sarcoma.
Antimicrotubule agents	Inhibits microtubule function that disrupts mitotic and non-mitotic cell function.	Vincristine: leukemia, lymphoma. Vinorelbine: lung, breast cancer. Paclitaxel: lung, breast, bladder cancer.
Miscellaneous	Inhibits protein synthesis: DNA demethylation agent: Inhibits histone deacetylase:	L-aspariginase: acute lymphoblastic leukemia. 5-azacitidine: myelodysplastic syndrome. Bortezomib: multiple myeloma

4

What You Can Do

The spiritual power of Eastern practices linked to the scientific rigor of Western medical research is a potent remedy. Eastern modalities such as yoga, acupuncture, and meditation have been scientifically shown to increase circulating T cells, the white blood cells that destroy cancer cells. This means that, whatever tumor removal, tumor destruction, or immunological treatments your oncologist may prescribe, they can be supplemented by Eastern spiritual practices. This includes other activities such as exercise, joy, optimism, massage, or a good evening out with friends. In other words, a large part of the cure of your cancer is in your hands, assuming you want to survive.

Descriptions of Yoga, acupuncture, meditation, exercise, and other healing modalities were a part of the first edition of *The Key to Cancer*. However, they are now so widely accepted and practiced I feel they no longer need be described by me. But, be very sure, a combination of them is vital to good physical, emotional and spiritual health.

And, coincidentally, attention to the role of these "supplemental modalities" does clarify the previously unexplained phenomena of "spontaneous remission" and "delayed recurrence" that periodically occur in cancer patients.

5

Where to from Here?

We can keep it simple, and get it wrong, or deal with its complexity and get it right. The cure of cancer consists of both removing tumor as well as repairing the injured protective complex which permitted the tumor to develop in the first place.

So where does this leave you, the cancer patient? We hope with a lot of useful information. But how about the follow-up? I recommend each patient make up a "self-prescription for health," in a form similar to the following. Each category should be filled in, but how depends on your age and capacities, hence **you** do it rather than someone else. Remember, when using any medication or supplement, to check it out with your oncologist so that it does not interfere with your tumor treatment.

SELF PRESCRIPTION

Exercise _____

Stress Management _____

Meditation/Yoga _____

Diet _____

Supplements _____

Relationships/Joy _____

Entertainment _____

Hobbies/Relaxation _____

Spiritual Practice _____

Giving to Others _____

Attitude/Psychological _____

You may need some help with this from a personal trainer, dietition, your oncologist, psychologist, and so on. But you should own your own program, otherwise it will be a duty imposed by others and probably doomed to failure. Most of all, plan to do something good for yourself every day: some exercise, a good book, dinner with a friend, a concert or play, a funny or heart-warming movie, a massage, whatever is worth looking forward to. Your enjoyment of life will help make you well.

1/2 MEASURES

Half a dose of CAM (complementary alternative medicine) therapy is no different than half a dose of chemotherapy, or surgical removal of half the tumor.

Please refer back to the apothecaries' scale in Chapter 1. This is a picture of cancer; implied in it is also the treatment. Now, on the left side of the balance there is, say, a five pound tumor. No one would suggest removing half of it surgically or by means of chemo or x-ray. That would be foolish. Equally foolish, however, is to add only two pounds to the already depleted right side, which may weigh in at only one or two pounds. In other words, CAM therapy must be as vigorous on the right side as tumor destruction (Western medicine) is on the left. Effectiveness on both sides is dose-related. And half measures on either side give the patient the false idea he is being adequately treated.

Now when is enough CAM therapy enough? There seems no measurable end point, but we have found the patient's energy level to be a useful guide. If you feel more energy than before, and this is stable (with the usual daily fluctuations) or increasing, you are doing well. Another index, of course, is evidence that your tumor is shrinking, either physically, by x-ray studies, or by improved tumor markers.

Whenever possible, we try to apply the same scientific standards for proof of results as is usual with medical oncology. Particularly in the area of spirit, this may be difficult, but we make a maximum effort.

The primary goal of this book has been to present a different conception of cancer. We hope we have succeeded. But we have a second motive, to make cancer education available to all, above and beyond this book. To gain that end, we have recently established a foundation for cancer education. Our mission statement follows:

Mission: We are a "school" devoted to cancer patients. We neither examine nor treat patients, leaving that to, and preferring to work with, the patients' own physicians. We do offer a comprehensive analysis of the four factors that contribute to cancer survival: conventional "Western" tumor destruction, further tumor control through the immune system, stimulation of energy which makes this possible, and emotional and spiritual support which enhances the patients' will to live.

Our foundation, The Richard Weeder Cancer Education Foundation, functions as an advisory organization for locally formed groups interested in instructing cancer patients, their care-givers, and other interested parties in how to approach the disease from a spiritual, emotional, and educational point of view. We provide, first, a core body of information, as found in *The Key to Cancer*. Second, we offer guidance in finding local practitioners of Eastern medicine and other healing modalities as instructors for a few-hours presentation of these modalities and other information from *The Key to Cancer*. We franchise, with modest affiliation cost, a program aimed to supplement and complement the Western information and drug-based therapy of oncology centers. Our approach has been validated at the highest level of medical oncology for its educational excellence. It is not "instead of" but "together with" the care the patient receives from reputable medical centers. With the exception of oncology, our instruction falls under our definition of protective therapy. Our program usually results in a life style change, but one that is generally pleasurable and (with the exception of oncology) carries little risk.

If further training or instruction beyond this book appeals to you, we suggest you find a hospital or health facility which offers both "Western" and "CAM" modalities. There are increasing numbers of them throughout the country. Or, if you prefer, you might find an individual or facility in your area who would wish to set up an affiliate program with ours. (See Affiliation/Collaboration.) We are prepared to facilitate programs at a distance. We will also facilitate study groups of as few as six patients, using this book as text, and audio or computer monitoring with an instructor from our staff or a qualified on-site practitioner from your area (R.N., M.D., D.O., or ND).

When searching for a therapist(s), we suggest finding one with the following credentials:

Acupuncture: *National:* Diplomate in Acupuncture
State: Lic.Ac or L.Ac (name of state)

Massage Therapy: State Licensure
National Certification (NCBMT)
AMTA membership—professional level

Oncology: Medical (chemotherapy): M.D. or D.O. and Boards in Hematology/Oncology
Radiation (X-ray): M.D. or D.O. and Boards in Radiation Therapy
Surgical: Fellow of American College of Surgeons, "Boarded," Fellowship in surgical oncology, etc.

Naturopathic Medicine: Postdoctoral board examination (NPLEX).
State Licensure

Exercise Therapy: A recommended "Personal Trainer" at a good gym. Credentials, training and experience working with cancer patients.

Yoga: See www.yogaalliance.org or, for special needs, www.viniyoga.com

Meditation: Check out centers at www.spiritrock.org, www.dharma.org and *Tricycle* magazine

Relational Therapy: Attitudinal Healing, Nonviolent Communication, Psychotherapy etc. See references in Bibliography.

*   *   *

A PREDICTION

In about twenty years the "state of the art" treatment of cancer will look like this:

1. Once the diagnosis of cancer is made, the medical (surgical, radiation and chemotherapy) oncologist will pursue a course of treatment as now, with the expected advances in their modalities, to obliterate tumor as far as possible.
2. In close collaboration with tumor removal, the Naturopathic Oncologist (or other trained CAM therapist) will support the immune system and energy stores which are damaged as a side effect of tumor destruction.
3. Following tumor removal, the protective therapist will orchestrate an intensive course of CAM therapy to bring back the right side of the scale and facilitate "mopping up" any residual nests of tumor left behind by western medicine.

4. The CAM therapist will then prescribe a maintenance program supporting immunity, energy and spirit to prevent recurrence or the development of new tumors. The conventional oncologist will follow the patient in tandem with the CAM oncologist.

5. Survival figures will be a lot better than they are now.

FAREWELL

With the above, you have equipped yourself with the most powerful healing tools of all: knowledge and hope. Congratulations, and be well.

6

Gratitude

I have known many who have given thanks for having had cancer. You most likely feel entirely differently. But let's put this into perspective.

Cancer may have caused you to rethink your priorities and your values. It may have brought you closer to friends and family or caused you to reestablish contact with someone important who had strayed away. It may have strengthened your faith, or shaken it. But at least it has probably caused to you to think deeply about the meaning of life and the essence of yourself as a human being.

There is a Bass aria in "Messiah" by Handel, "For He is like a refiner's fire," followed by the chorus, "And He shall purify the sons of Levi." You may have felt the pain of that fire, but you may also have been purified. And for that, feel grateful, for gratitude is itself healing.

It's all in the point of view. We have considered cancer not the cause of disease, but the effect of a lapse in the healing mechanisms that protect us. So be confident that, by strengthening those mechanisms, you will be healthier than you were before, in so many ways.

We will not bless you. Only yourself, or a higher power, can do that. But we salute you.

Aloha.

7

Epilogue:
The Question of Proof

We have not proven our thesis of causality beyond all doubt, nor that the "protective complex" can either prevent or cure cancer. What we have laid out is a body of evidence, some of which depends on the reader's own experience. For how many of us have **not** seen a patient who has undergone a spontaneous, unexplained and unexpected remission. These are, admittedly, anecdotes. But laid end to end, enough anecdotes become "clinical experience."

For thirty-five years, ever since I began working with cancer, I have tried to figure it out. With other conditions, such as appendicitis, I could detail to myself, my patients and my students the cause, pathology, anatomy and physiology. There was a logical progression of the disease which made sense, and an operation which successfully stopped the downhill course. But with cancer, it was a messy business—there were too many loose ends—until now. Not until I took the causality to a deeper level did the pieces of the puzzle start to fall into place.

In order to write the last chapter of this book, we will need five years and experience with five hundred patients. But in the meantime, enough evidence is in to know what the message is. And there are a lot of people who don't have five years to wait for our answer.

With regard to other proofs, such as the statements that massage and exercise increase immunity, or that exercise and nutrition increase energy, or that relationships and faith increase will to live, there is ample evidence in the literature. And there is no scientific standard by which to measure a partly philosophic treatise. Finally, the only person who needs persuading is you, the reader. If there is the ring of truth in what we have said, we are pleased. The law has an expression for it: *Res ipsa loquitur,* the thing speaks for itself.

8

Affiliation/Collaboration

The Richard Weeder Cancer Education Foundation invites affiliation or collaboration with our program by groups of health care providers interested in educating the cancer patient. The following guidelines apply.

1) Programs are locally organized and run, under the supervision of a health care professional.

2) Affiliation or collaboration would require that the program be broad-based, with educators from the following modalities, or their equivalents: Medical, radiation or surgical oncology; Exercise therapy; Nutrition (including immunity, antioxidants, and supplements); Meditation; Yoga, Tai Chi or equivalent; Acupuncture; Massage therapy; Relationship therapy (Nonviolent Communication, Attitudinal Healing, Psychotherapy or equivalent); and nonsectarian religious or spiritual techniques.

3) All teachers are well-credentialed in their specialties.

4) Collaboration status would include affiliation but would go beyond it to include the sharing of patient data.

5) Affiliation or Collaboration status can and will be acknowledged on any brochures, advertisements or

literature you use in your program.

6) We will furnish advice and printed materials during the organizational phase and follow up during a collaborative arrangement, including a consent for study, letters to be sent to referring doctors, etc.

The program has been judged exempt from Institutional Review Board supervision as it is purely educational and no patient identification is made.

Nominal fees will be charged, primarily for secretarial and communication expenses. If personal assistance in the way of lectures and participation in the seminars is desired, that can also be arranged with Dr. Weeder or a faculty member at additional charge.

Follow-up non-organ-specific support groups in your locality are encouraged.

The Richard Weeder Cancer
Education Foundation

Bibliography

A Course in Miracles. Foundation for Inner Peace, Inc. 1975

Bock, Kenneth, and Sabin, Nellie. *The Road To Immunity*. New York: Pocket Books. 1997

Bovbjerg, D. H. and Valdimarsdottir, H. B. "Psychoneuroimmunology: Implications for Psychooncology". In Holland, J. C. *Psycho-oncology* Oxford: Oxford Univ. Press. 2001

Conrad, Joseph. *Lord Jim*. New York: Dell Publishing Co., Inc. 1961

Dickens, Charles. *A Christmas Carol*

Dossey, Larry. *Healing Words*. New York: Harper Collins. 1993

Dossey, Larry. *What's Love Got to do With It*. Alternative Therapies May 1996. Vol. 2. No. 3

Easwaran, Eknath. *Conquest of Mind*. Tomales, CA: Nilgiri Press. 1988

Hendrix, Harville. *Getting the Love You Want*. New York Henry Holt & Co. 1988

Jampolsky, Gerald G. *Forgiveness: The Greatest Healer of All*. Hillsboro OR: Beyond Words Pub. 1999

Nhat Hahn, Thich. *The Miracle of Mindfulness*. Boston: Beacon Press. 1975

Ornish, Dean. *Dr. Dean Ornish's Program for Reversing Heart Disease*. N Y Random House. 1990

Pelletier, Kenneth R. *The Best Alternative Medicine*. New York: Simon and
    Schuster. 2000

Rosenberg, Marshall B. *Nonviolent Communication: A Language of Life*.
    Encinitas, Ca. Puddledancer Press. 2003

Seligman, Martin. E. P. *Learned Optimism*. New York: Pocket Books. 1990

Simonton, O. Carl, Mathews-Simonton, Stephanie, and Creighton, James L.
    Getting Well Again. New York: Bantam books. 1980

Specter, Michael. "The Outlaw Doctor" In *The New Yorker*, Feb. 5, 2001
    (Article on Nicholas Gonzales, M.D.)

Tolle, Eckhart. *Practicing the Power of Now*. Novato, California: New World
    Library. 1999

Wallace, R. K. and Benson, H. "The Physiology of Meditation" *Scientific
    American*. Vol. 19: 226: 1972 pp. 84–90 1972

Weeder, Richard S., Zunin, Ira, Okazaki, Ian, Lurie, Fedor. "The Educational
    Approach to Advanced Cancer: A Preliminary Report." *Hawaii Medical
    Journal*, Nov., 2005; 64: 305–306.

Weil, Andrew. "Sound Body. Sound Mind." Compact Disc. New York: Upaya,
    Division of Music. 1997

Weil, Andrew. "Self Healing. Creating Natural Health for your Body and
    Mind." (Monthly Newsletter) Watertown, Mass.

To contact us or buy more books by Dr. Weeder:
www.richardweeder.com
or
shop@richardweeder.com